Quick and Sweet: Bread Machine Cookbook

50 easy and affordable quick and sweet recipes for your bread machine

Raul Wyatt

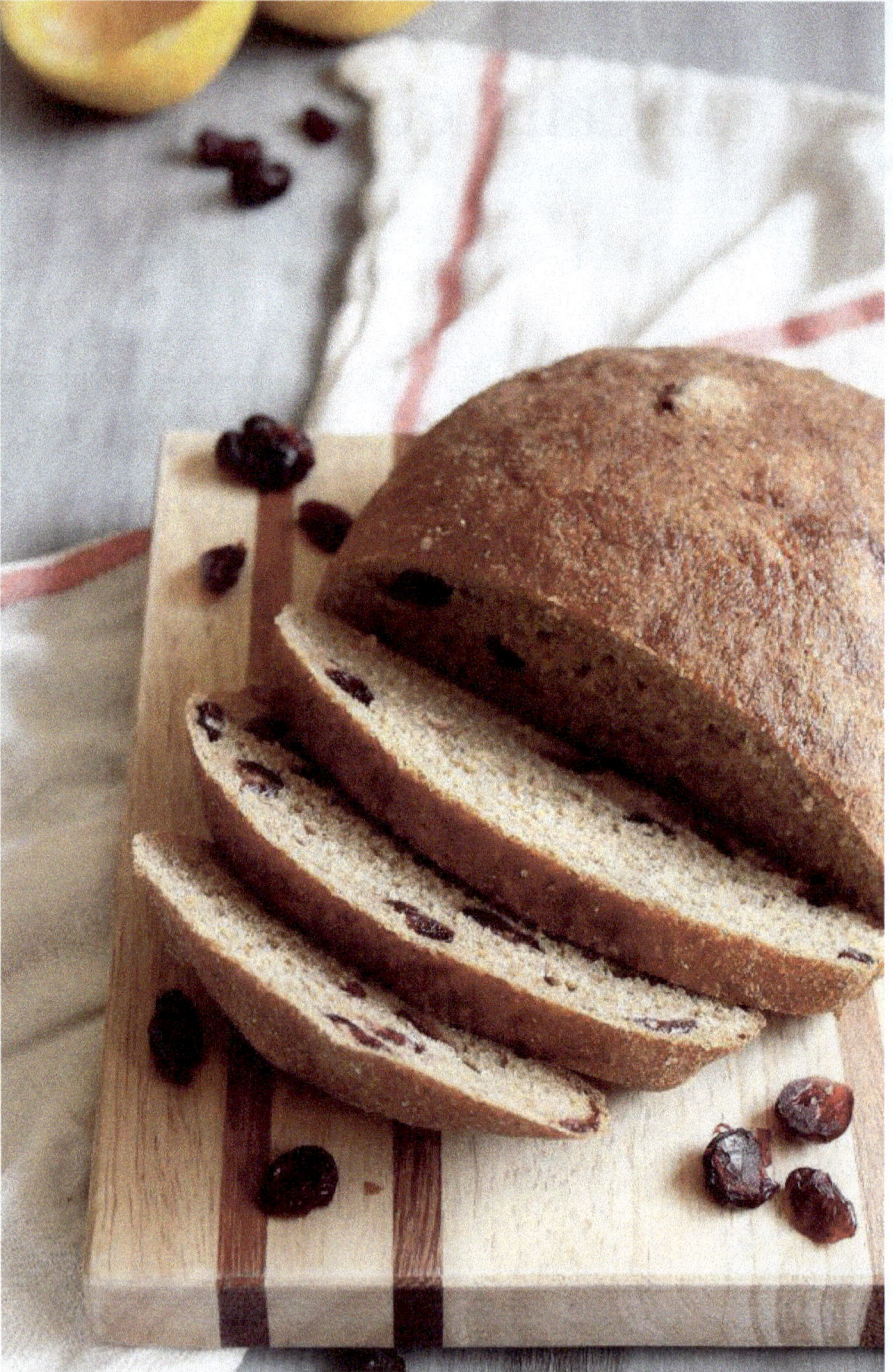

COPYRIGHT

Table of Contents

Egg Bread

Preparation Time: 10 minutes

1½-Pound Loaf

Ingredients:

· 4 cups bread flour, sifted

· 1 cup lukewarm milk

· 2 whole eggs

· 1 teaspoon active dry yeast

· 1½ teaspoons salt

· 2¼ tablespoons white sugar

· 1½ tablespoons butter, melted

Directions:

1.Prepare all of the ingredients for your bread and measuring means (a cup, a spoon, kitchen scales).

2.Carefully measure the ingredients into the pan.

3.Put all the ingredients into a bread bucket in the right order, follow your manual for the bread machine.

4.Close the cover. Select the program of your bread machine to BASIC and choose the crust colour to MEDIUM.

5.Press START. Wait until the program completes.

6.When done, take the bucket out and let it cool for 5 minutes.

7.Shake the pound from the pan and let cool for 30 minutes on a cooling rack.

8.Slice, serve, and enjoy the taste of fragrant homemade bread.

Nutrition:

· Calories: 319

· Fat: 5.6 g

· Cholesterol: 56 g

· Sodium: 365 mg

· Carbohydrates: 56.7 g

· Fiber: 1.1 g

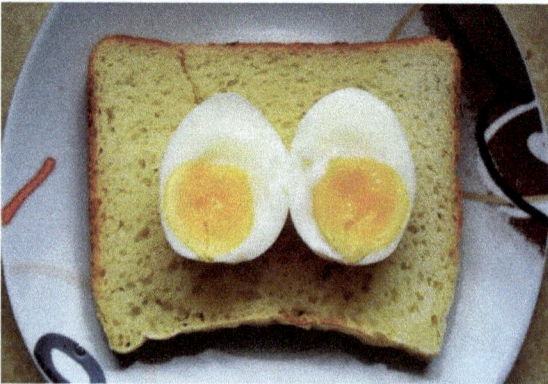

Honey Pound Cake

Preparation Time: 10 minutes

1-Pound Loa

Ingredients:

· 1 cup butter, unsalted

· ½ cup water

· ¼ cup honey

· 2 tablespoons whole milk

· 4 eggs, beaten

· 1 cup of sugar

· 2 cups flour

· Pinch of salt

Directions:

1.Bring the butter to room temperature and cut into ½ -inch cubes.

2.Add all ingredients to the bread machine in the order listed (butter, honey, milk, eggs, sugar, flour).

3. Press Sweetbread setting follow by light crust colour, then press Start. Take out the cake on the bread pan using a rubber

spatula as soon as it's finished. Cool on a rack and serve with your favorite fruit.

Nutrition:

· Calories: 217

· Sodium: 33 mg

· Dietary Fiber: 0.3 g

· Fat: 6.9 g

· Carbohydrates: 13 g

· Protein: 1.9 g

Carrot Cake Bread

Preparation Time: 15 minutes

1-Pound Loaf

Ingredients:

· Non-stick cooking spray

· ¼ cup vegetable oil

· 2 large eggs, room temperature

· ½ teaspoon pure vanilla extract

· ½ cup sugar

· ¼ cup light brown sugar

· ¼ cup of crushed pineapple with juice (from a can or fresh)

· 5 cups unbleached, all-purpose flour

· 1 teaspoon baking powder

· ¼ teaspoon baking soda

· ¼ teaspoon salt

· 1 teaspoon ground cloves

· ¾ teaspoon ground cinnamon

· 1 cup freshly grated carrots

· 1/3 cup chopped pecans

· 1/3 cup golden raisins

Directions:

1.Coat the inside of the bread pan with non-stick cooking spray.

2.Add all of the ingredients, in the order listed, to the bread pan.

3.Select Express Bake, medium crust colour, and press Start. While the batter is mixing

  scrape the bread pan's sides with a rubber spatula to incorporate ingredients fully.

4.When baked, remove from the bread pan and place on a wire rack to cool completely before slicing and serving.

Nutrition:

· Calories: 181

· Sodium: 60 mg

· Protein: 2,4g

· Dietary Fiber: 1.2 g

· Fat: 7.2 g

· Carbohydrates: 11 g

Lemon Cake

Preparation Time: 10 minutes

1 ½-Pound Loaf

Ingredients:

· 3 large eggs, beaten

· 1/3 cup milk

· ½ cup butter, melted

· 2 cups all-purpose flour

· 3 teaspoons baking powder

· 1 1/3 cups sugar

· 1 teaspoon vanilla extract

· 2 lemons, zested

· For the glaze:

· 1 cup powdered sugar

· 2 tablespoons lemon juice, freshly squeezed

Directions:

1.Prepare the glaze by whisking the powder sugar and lemon juice together in a small mixing bowl and set aside.

2.Add all remaining ingredients to the baking pan in the order listed.

3.Select the Sweetbread, medium colour crust, and press Start.

4.When baked, transfer the baking pan to a cooling rack.

5.When the cake has cooled, gently shake the cake out into a serving plate. Glaze the cold cake and serve.

Nutrition:

· Calories: 290

· Sodium: 77 mg

· Dietary Fiber: 0.6 g

· Fat: 9.3 g

· Carbohydrates: 42.9 g

· Protein: 4 g.

Insane Coffee Cake

Preparation Time: 25 minutes

3-Pound Loaf

Ingredients:

· 7 cups of milk

· ¼ cup of sugar

· 1 teaspoon salt

· 1 egg yolk

· 1 tablespoon butter

· 2¼ cups bread flour

· 2 teaspoons of active dry yeast

For the topping:

· 2 tablespoons butter, melted

· 2 tablespoons brown sugar

· 1 teaspoon cinnamon

Directions:

1.Set the topping ingredients set aside, then add the other ingredients to the bread pan in the order above.

2.Set the bread machine to the Dough process.

3.Butter a 9-by-9-inch glass baking dish and pour the dough into the container. Cover with a towel and rise for about 5minutes.

4. Preheat an oven to 375° F.

5.Brush the dough with the melted butter.

6.Put brown sugar and cinnamon in a bowl, mix it well, and then put a sprinkle on top of the coffee cake.

7.Let the topped dough rise, uncovered, for another 30 minutes.

8.Place in oven and bake for 35 minutes or until a wooden toothpick inserted into the center comes out clean and dry.

9.When baked, let the coffee cake rest for 5minutes. Carefully remove the coffee cake from the dish with a rubber spatula, slice, and serve.

Nutrition:

· Calories: 211

· Sodium: 240 mg

· Dietary Fiber: 0.9 g

· Fat: 3.9 g

· Carbohydrates: 24.9 g

· Protein: 3.5 g

Chocolate Marble Cake

Preparation Time: 25 minutes

1½-Pounds Loaf

Ingredients:

· 1½ cups water

· 1½ teaspoons vanilla extract

· 1½ teaspoons salt

· 3½ cups bread flour

· 1½ teaspoons instant yeast

· 1 cup semi-sweet chocolate chips

Directions:

1.Set the chocolate chips aside and add the other ingredients to your bread maker's pan.

2.Program the machine for Sweetbread and then press Start.

3.Check the dough after 15 minutes of kneading, you should have a smooth ball, soft but not sticky.

4.Add the chocolate chips about 3 minutes before the end of the second kneading cycle.

5.Cool on a rack before serving.

Pumpkin Spice Cake

Preparation Time: 10 minutes

1½ pound Loaf

Ingredients:

· 1 cup of sugar

· 1 cup canned pumpkin

· 1/3 cup vegetable oil

· 1 teaspoon vanilla extract

· 2 eggs

· 1 ½ cups all-purpose flour

· 2 teaspoons baking powder

· ¼ teaspoon salt

· 1 teaspoon ground cinnamon

· ¼ teaspoon ground nutmeg

· 1½ teaspoons ground cloves

· Shortening, for greasing pan

Directions:

1.Grease bread maker pan and kneading blade generously with shortening.

2.Add all ingredients to the pan in the order listed above.

3.Select the Rapid cycle and press Start.

4. Open the lid three minutes into the cycle,

5.Carefully scrape the pan's downsides with a rubber spatula, close the lid to continue the process.

6.Cool the baked cake for 5minutes on a wire rack before slicing.

Nutrition:

· Calories: 245

· Sodium: 46 mg

· Dietary Fiber: 1.3 g

· Fat: 7.1 g

· Carbohydrates: 31.2 g

· Protein: 2.1 g

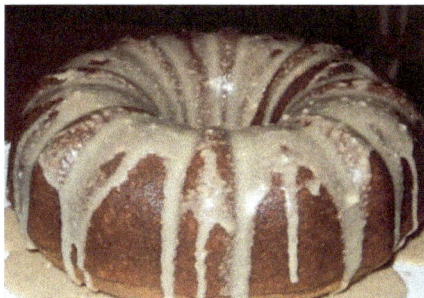

Lemon Blueberry Quick Bread

Preparation Time: 1 hour

1¼-Pound Loaf

Ingredients:

· 2 cups all-purpose flour

· 1½ teaspoons baking powder

· ½ teaspoon salt

· 1 tablespoon lemon zest

· 1 cup of sugar

· ½ cup unsalted butter, softened

· 2 large eggs

· 2 teaspoons pure vanilla extract

· ½ cup whole milk

· 1½ cups blueberries

For the crumb topping:

· 1/3 cup sugar

· 3 tablespoons all-purpose flour

· 2 tablespoons butter, melted

· Non-stick cooking spray

Directions:

1.Spray bread maker pan with non-stick cooking spray and lightly flour.

2.Combine crumb topping ingredients and set aside.

3.In a small bowl, put the whisk together with flour, baking powder, and salt and set aside.

4.In a large bowl, put the sugar and lemon zest, then mix them. Add butter and beat until light and fluffy. Add eggs, vanilla, and milk.

5.Add flour mixture and mix until combined. Stir in blueberries and spread batter evenly into bread maker pan.

6.Top with crumb topping, select Sweetbread, light colour crust, and press Start.

7. When the cake is made, cool it on a wire rack for 15 minutes and serves warm.

Nutrition:

· Calories: 462

· Sodium: 120 mg

· Dietary Fiber: 1 g

· Fat: 32.1 g

· Carbohydrates: 41.1 g

· Protein: 4 g

Cinnamon Pecan Coffee Cake

Preparation Time: 1 hour

2-Pound Loaf

Ingredients:

· 1 cup butter, unsalted

· 1 cup of sugar

· 2 eggs

· 1 cup sour cream

· 1 teaspoon vanilla extract

· 2 cups all-purpose flour

· 1 teaspoon baking powder

· 1 teaspoon baking soda

· ½ teaspoon salt

For the topping:

· ½ cup brown sugar

· ¼ cup sugar

· ½ cup pecans, chopped

· ½ teaspoon cinnamon

Directions:

1.Add butter, sugar, eggs, sour cream, and vanilla to the bread maker baking pan, followed by the dry ingredients.

2. Select the Cake cycle and press Start, then Prepare toppings and set aside.

3.When the kneading cycle is done, about1 minute, sprinkle 1/2 cup of topping on top of the dough and continue baking.

4.During the last hour of baking time, sprinkle the remaining 1/2 cup of topping on the cake. Bake until complete. Cool it on a wire rack for 5minutes and serve warm.

Nutrition:

· Calories: 411

· Carbohydrates: 10 g

· Sodium: 120 mg

· Fiber: 2.5 g

· Fat: 32.1 g

Whole Wheat Bread

Preparation Time: 15 minutes

Ingredients:

> 1-Pound
>
> 1 ½-Pound
>
> 2-Pound

Lukewarm whole milk

> ½ cup
>
> 1 cup
>
> 11/3 cups

Unsalted butter, diced

> 2 tablespoons
>
> 3 tablespoons
>
> 4 tablespoons

Whole wheat flour

1 cup

1½ cups

2 cups

Plain bread flour

1 cup

1½ cups

2 cups

Brown sugar

2 ½ tablespoons

3 ¾ tablespoons

5 tablespoons

Salt

¾ teaspoon

1¼ teaspoons

1½ teaspoons

Bread machine yeast

¾ teaspoon

1¼ teaspoons

1½ teaspoons

Directions:

1.Add the ingredients into the bread machine as per the order of the ingredients listed above or follow your bread machine's instruction manual.

2.Select the whole wheat setting and medium crust function.

3.When ready, turn the bread out onto a drying rack and allow it to cool, then serve.

Tip(s):

1.After the bread has kneaded for the first time, sprinkle oats or seeds over the top and then allow the machine to continue baking.

Nutrition:

· Calories: 231

· Total fat: 3.2 g

· Saturated fat: 1.1½ g

· Cholesterol: 1½ mg

· carbohydrates: 22.9 g

· Dietary fiber: 2.1 g

· Sodium: 139 mg

Whole Wheat and Honey Bread

Preparation Time: 10 minutes

Ingredients:

    1-Pound

    1½-Pound

    2-Pound

Lukewarm water

    1 cup

    1½ cups

    2¼ cups

Honey

    3 tablespoons

    4½ tablespoon s

    6 tablespoons

Vegetable oil

    2 tablespoons

    3 tablespoons

    4 tablespoons

Plain bread flour

1½ cup

2 ¼ cups

3 cups

Whole wheat flour

1½ cups

2 ¼ cups

3 cups

Salt

1/3 teaspoon

¼ teaspoon

½ teaspoon

Instant dry yeast

1½ teaspoons

2¼ teaspoons

3 teaspoons

Directions:

1.Add the ingredients into the bread machine as per the order of the ingredients listed above or follow your bread machine's instruction manual.

2.Select the whole wheat setting and medium crust function.

3.When ready, turn the bread out onto a drying rack and allow it to cool, then serve.

Tip(s):

1.When the bread is ready, glaze the top with honey and add a few sesame seeds or rolled oats.

Nutrition:

· Calories: 210

· Total fat: 3.5 g

· Saturated fat: 0 g

· Cholesterol: 0 mg

· Total carbohydrates: 33.4 g

· Dietary fiber: 2.1 ½ g

· Sodium: 79 mg

· Protein: 5.2 g

100% Whole Wheat Bread

Preparation Time: 10 minutes

Ingredients:

    1-Pound

    1 ½-Pound

    2-Pound

Lukewarm water

    1 cup

    1 ½ cups

    2 cups

Milk powder

    1¼ tablespoons

    2 tablespoons

    2½ tablespoons

Unsalted butter, diced

    1 tablespoon

    1½ tablespoons

    2½ tablespoons

Honey

1 tablespoon

1½ tablespoons

2½ tablespoons

Molasses

1tablespoon

2 tablespoons

2½ tablespoons

Salt

1 teaspoon

1½ teaspoons

2 teaspoons

Whole wheat flour

2¼ cups

31/3 cups

4½ cups

Active dry yeast

1 teaspoon

1 ½ teaspoon

2 teaspoons

Directions:

1.Add the ingredients into the bread machine as per the order of the ingredients listed above or follow your bread machine's instruction manual.

2.Select the whole wheat setting and medium crust function.

3.When ready, turn the bread out onto a drying rack and allow it to cool, then serve.

Tip(s):

1.I combine the milk powder and water before adding them to the bread machine.

Nutrition:

· Calories: 229

· Total fat: 1 g

· Saturated fat: 0.5 g

· Cholesterol: 1.9 mg

· Carbohydrates: 30.4 g

· Dietary fiber: 0.9 g

· Sodium: 160 mg

· Protein: 4.0 g

Seeded Whole Wheat Bread

Preparation Time: 10 minutes

Ingredients:

    1-Pound

    1½-Pound

    2-Pound

Lukewarm water

    2/3cup

    1 cup

    ¼ cups

Milk powder

    3 tablespoons

    4½ tablespoons

    6 tablespoons

Honey

    1 tablespoon

    1½ tablespoons

    2 tablespoons

Unsalted butter, softened

 1 tablespoon

 1½ tablespoons

 2 tablespoons

Plain bread flour

 1 cup

 1½ cups

 2 cups

Whole wheat flour

 1 cup

 1½ cups

 2 cups

Poppy seeds

 2 tablespoons

 3 tablespoons

 4 tablespoons

Sesame seeds

 2 tablespoons

 3 tablespoons

 4 tablespoons

Sunflower seeds

2 tablespoons

3 tablespoons

4 tablespoons

Salt

¾ teaspoon

1 teaspoon

1½ teaspoons

Instant dry yeast

2 teaspoons

3 teaspoons

4 teaspoons

Directions:

1.Add the ingredients into the bread machine as per the order of the ingredients listed above or follow your bread machine's instruction manual.

2.Select the basic setting and medium crust function.

3.When ready, turn the bread out onto a drying rack and allow it to cool, then serve.

Tip(s):

1.Feel free to make use of any fine seeds, such as pumpkin or sesame seeds.

Nutrition:

· Calories: 240

· Total fat: 2 g

· Saturated fat: 1 g

· Cholesterol: 2 mg

· Carbohydrates: 1 g

· Dietary fiber: 1 g

· Sodium: 133 mg

· Protein: 3 g

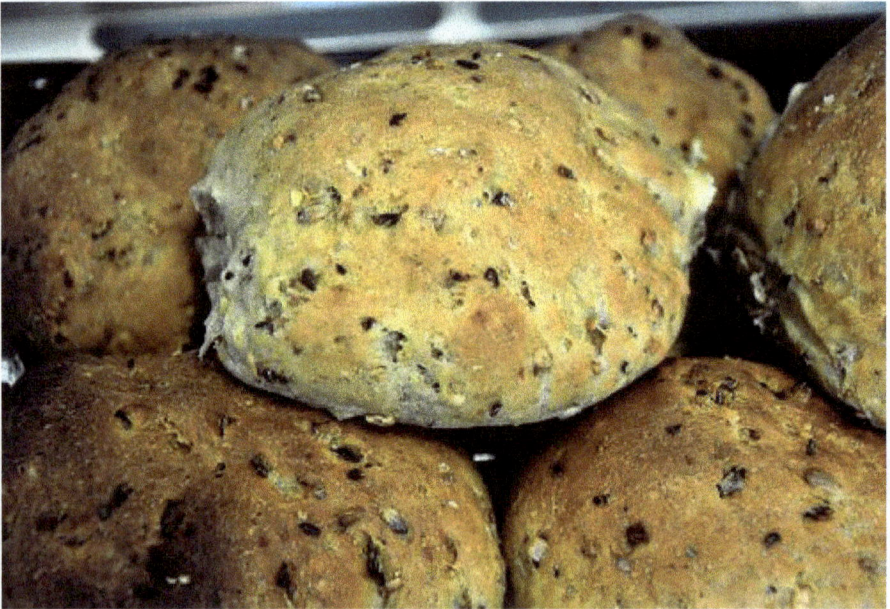

French Ham Bread

Preparation Time: 45 minutes

1½-Pound Loaf

Ingredients:

· 3 1/3 cups wheat flour

· 1 cup ham

· ½ cup of milk powder

· 1½ tablespoons sugar

· 1 teaspoon yeast, fresh

· 1 teaspoon salt

· 1 teaspoon dried basil

· 11/3 cups water

· 2 tablespoons olive oil

Directions:

1.Cut ham into cubes of 0.5-1 cm (approximately ¼ inch).

2.Put all ingredients in the bread maker from the following order: water, olive oil, salt, sugar, flour, milk powder, ham, and yeast.

3.Put all the ingredients according to the instructions in your bread maker.

4.Basil put in a dispenser or fill it later, at the signal in the container.

5. Turn on the bread maker.

6.After the end of the baking cycle, leave the bread container in the bread maker to keep warm for 1 hour.

7.Then your delicious bread is ready!

Nutrition:

· Calories: 210

· Total Fat: 5.5g

· Saturated Fat: 1.1 g

· Cholesterol: 1g

· Sodium: 240 mg

· Carbohydrates: 47.2 g

· Dietary Fiber: 1.7 g

· Sugars: 6.4 g

· Protein: 11.4 g

Meat Bread

Preparation Time: 1 hour

1½-Pound Loaf

Ingredients:

· 2 cups boiled chicken

· 1 cup milk

· 3 cups flour

· 1 tablespoon dry yeast

· 1 egg

· 1 teaspoon sugar

· ½ tablespoon salt

· 2 tablespoons oil

Directions:

1.Pre-cook the meat. You can use a leg or fillet.

2.Separate meat from the bone and cut it into small pieces.

3.Pour all ingredients into the bread maker according to the instructions.

4.Add chicken pieces now.

5.The program is Basic.

6.This bread is perfectly combined with dill and butter.

Nutrition:

· Calories: 210

· Total Fat: 6.2 g

· Saturated Fat: 1.4 g

· Cholesterol: 50 g

· Sodium: 120 mg

· Carbohydrates: 31g

· Dietary Fiber: 1.6g

· Sugars: 2g

· Protein: 17.2g

Fish Bell Pepper Bran Bread

Preparation Time: 1 hour

1 ½-Pound Loaf

Ingredients:

· 2½ cups flour

· ½ cup bran

· 1 1/3 cups water

· 1½ teaspoons salt

· 1½ teaspoons sugar

· 1½ tablespoons mustard oil

· 1¼ teaspoons dry yeast

· 2 teaspoons powdered milk

· 1 cup chopped bell pepper

· ¾ cup chopped smoked fish

· 1 onion

Directions:

1. Grind onion and fry until golden brown.

2.Cut the fish into small pieces and the pepper into cubes.

3.Load all the ingredients in the bucket.

4.Turn on the baking program.

Bon Appetit!

Nutrition:

· Calories: 210

· Total Fat 3.1 ½ g

· Saturated Fat: 0.5 g

· Cholesterol: 1 ½ g

· Sodium: 411mg

· Carbohydrates: 35.9 g

· Dietary Fiber: 4.2 g

· Sugars: 2.7 g

· Protein: 7.2 g

Sausage Bread

Preparation Time: 20 minutes

1 ½-Pound Loaf

Ingredients:

· 1½ teaspoons dry yeast

· 3 cups flour

· 1 teaspoon sugar

· 1½ teaspoons salt

· 11/3 cups whey

· 1 tablespoon oil

· 1 cup chopped smoked sausage

Directions:

1.Fold all the ingredients in the order that is recommended specifically for your model.

2.Set the required parameters for baking bread.

3.When ready, remove the delicious hot bread.

4.Wait until it cools down and enjoy sausage.

Nutrition:

· Calories: 234

· Total Fat 5.1 g

· Saturated Fat: 1.2 g

· Cholesterol: 9 g

· Sodium: 435 mg

· Carbohydrates: 31 g

· Dietary Fiber: 1.4 g

· Sugars: 2.7 g

· Protein: 7.4 g

Cheese Sausage Bread

Preparation Time: 20 minutes

1 ½-Pound Loaf

Ingredients

· 1 teaspoon dry yeast

· 3½ cups flour

· 1 teaspoon salt

· 1 tablespoon sugar

· 1½ tablespoons oil

· 2 tablespoons smoked sausage

· 2 tablespoons grated cheese

· 1 tablespoon chopped garlic

· 1 cup of water

Directions:

1. Cut the sausage into small cubes.

2. Grate the cheese on a grater

3. Chop the garlic.

4.Add all ingredients to the machine according to the instructions.

5.Turn on the baking program, and let it do the work.

Nutrition:

· Calories: 260

· Total Fat 5.6 g

· Saturated Fat: 1.4 g

· Cholesterol: 1½ g

· Sodium: 355 mg

· Carbohydrates: 43 g

· Dietary Fiber: 1.6 g

· Sugars: 1.7 g

· Protein: 7.7 g

Cheesy Pizza Dough

Preparation Time: 1 Hour

Servings: 4

Ingredients:

· ½ cup warm beer, or more as needed

· 1 tablespoon Parmesan cheese

· 1½ teaspoons pizza dough yeast

· 1 teaspoon salt

· 1 teaspoon ground black pepper

· 1 teaspoon granulated garlic

· 1 tablespoon olive oil

· 5 cups of all-purpose flour, or more if needed

Directions:

1.In a big mixing bowl, mix granulated garlic, pepper, salt, yeast, Parmesan cheese, and beer. Mix until salt dissolves. Allow mixture to stand for 4 minutes until yeast creates a creamy layer. Mix in olive oil.

2.Mix flour in yeast mixture until dough becomes smooth. Add small amounts of flour or beer if the dough is too sticky or dry.

Let rise for an hour. Punch the dough and roll into a pizza crust on a work surface that's floured.

Nutrition:

· Calories: 199

· Carbohydrates: 32 g

· Cholesterol: 1 mg

· Total Fat: 4.2 g

· Protein: 5.4 g

· Sodium: 330 mg

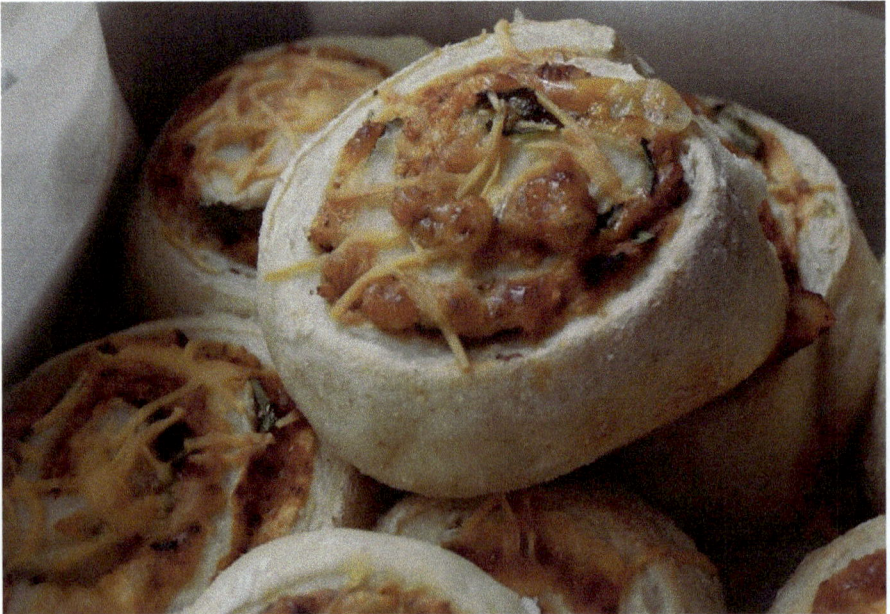

Collards & Bacon Grilled Pizza

Preparation Time: 15 minutes

Servings: 4

Ingredients:

· 1 lb. whole-wheat pizza dough

· 3 tablespoons garlic-flavoured olive oil

· 2 cups thinly sliced cooked collard greens

· 1 cup shredded Cheddar cheese

· ¼ cup crumbled cooked bacon

Directions:

1.Heat grill to medium-high.

2.Roll out dough to an oval that's 1 ½ inches on a surface that's lightly floured. Move to a big baking sheet that's lightly floured. Put Cheddar, collards, oil, and dough on the grill.

3.Grease grill rack. Move to grill the crust. Cover the lid and cook for 1-2 minutes until it becomes light brown and puffed. Use tongs to flip over the crust—spread oil on the crust and top with Cheddar and collards. Close lid and cook until cheese melts for another 2-3 minutes or the crust is light brown at the bottom.

4.Put pizza on the baking sheet and top using bacon.

Nutrition:

· Calories: 491

· Carbohydrates: 50 g

· Cholesterol: 33 mg

· Total Fat: 21 ½ g

· Fiber: 6 g

· Protein: 19 g

· Sodium: 573 mg

· Sugar: 3 g

Deep Dish Pizza Dough

Preparation Time: 25 minutes

Servings: 1½

Ingredients:

· 1 package active dry yeast

· 1/3 cup white sugar

· 2/3 cup water

· 2 cups all-purpose flour

· 1 cup bread flour

· ¼ cup corn oil

· 2 teaspoons salt

· 6 tablespoons vegetable oil

· ½ cup all-purpose flour, or if it's needed

Directions:

1.Dissolve sugar and yeast in a bowl with water. Stand the mixture for 5 minutes until the yeast starts to form creamy foam and softens.

2.In a bowl, mix bread flour, salt, corn oil, and 2 cups of all-purpose flour. Add the yeast mixture. Knead the mixture on a work surface using 1/2 of the all-purpose flour until well-incorporated. Place the dough in a warm area, then rise for 2 hours until its size doubles.

Nutrition:

· Calories: 321

· Carbohydrate: 31 g

· Cholesterol: 0 mg

· Total Fat: 17.5 g

· Protein: 4.4 g

· Sodium: 511 mg

Double Crust Stuffed Pizza

Preparation Time: 1 hour

1 ½-Pound Loaf

Ingredients:

· 1½ teaspoons white sugar

· 1 cup of warm water

· 1½ teaspoons active dry yeast

· 1 tablespoon olive oil

· 1½ teaspoons salt

· 2 cups all-purpose flour

· 1 can crushed tomatoes

· 1 tablespoon packed brown sugar

· ½ teaspoon garlic powder

· 1 teaspoon olive oil

· 3 cups shredded mozzarella cheese, divided

· ½ lb. bulk Italian sausage

· 1 package sliced pepperoni

· 1 package sliced fresh mushrooms

· ½ green bell pepper, chopped

· ½ red bell pepper, chopped

Directions:

1. In a large bowl or work bowl of a stand mixer, mix warm water and white sugar. Sprinkle with yeast and let the mixture stand for 5 minutes until the yeast starts to form creamy foam and softens. Stir in 1 tbsp. Of olive oil.

2. Mix flour with ½ teaspoon. of salt. Add half flour mixture into the yeast mixture and mix until no dry spots are visible. Whisk in remaining flour, a half cup at a time, mixing well every after addition. Put the dough on a lightly floured surface once it has pulled together. Knead the dough for 1 ½ minutes until elastic and smooth. You can use the dough hook in a stand mixer to mix it.

3. Transfer it into a lightly oiled bowl and flip to coat the dough with oil. Use a light cloth to cover the dough. Rise it in a warm place for 1 hour until the volume doubles.

4. In a small saucepan, mix 1 tsp of olive oil, brown sugar, crushed tomatoes, garlic powder, and salt. Cover the saucepan and let it cook in low heat for 30 minutes until the tomatoes begin to break down.

5. Set the oven to 450°F for preheating. Flatten the dough and place it on a lightly floured surface. Divide the dough into two equal portions. Roll one part into a 1 ½ -inches thin circle, then Roll the other piece into a 9-inches thicker circle.

6. Press the ½ -inches dough round into an ungreased 9-inches springform pan. Top the dough with a cup of cheese. Form sausage into a 9-inches patty and place it on top of the cheese.

Arrange the pepperoni, green pepper, mushrooms, red pepper, and the remaining cheese on top of the sausage patty. Place the 9-inches dough around on the top, pinching its edges to seal. Make vent holes on the top of the crust by cutting several ½ - inch. Pour the sauce evenly on the crust, leaving an only ½ -inch border at the edges.

7.Bake the pizza inside the preheated oven for 40-45 minutes until the cheese is melted, then check sausage is cooked through when the crust is fixed. Let the pizza rest for 15 minutes. Before serving, cut the pizza into wedges.

Nutrition:

· Calories: 250

· Carbohydrates: 32 g

· Fat: 21.1 g

· Protein: 22.2 g

· Sodium: 350 mg

French Crusty Loaf Bread

Preparation Time: 20 minutes

2-Pound Loaf

Ingredients:

· 5 slices bread

· 2 cups + 2 tablespoons water, lukewarm

· 4 teaspoons sugar

· 2 teaspoons table salt

· 6½ cups white bread flour

· 2 teaspoons bread machine yeast

· 1½ slices bread (1 ½ pound)

· 1½ cups + 1 tablespoon water, lukewarm between 1 1/1 and 90 º F

· 3 teaspoons sugar

· 1½ teaspoons table salt

· 4¾ cups white bread flour

· 1½ teaspoons bread machine yeast

Directions:

1.Choose the size of pound you would like to make and measure your ingredients.

2.Put the ingredients to the bread pan in the order list above.

3. Place the pan in the machine and close the lid.

4.Switch on the bread maker. Select the French setting, then the pound size, and finally, the crust colour. Start the cycle.

5.When the process is finished and the bread is baked, remove the pan from the machine. Use a potholder as the handle. Rest for a few minutes.

6.Take out the bread from the pan and let it cool on a wire rack for at least 5 minutes before slicing.

Nutrition:

· Calories: 176

· Fat 1.2 g

· Carbohydrates: 31.4 g

· Sodium: 426 mg

· Protein: 5.7 g

Baguette Style French Bread

Preparation Time: 2 hours

2 Baguettes of 1 pound each

Ingredients for bread machine

· 1 2/3 cups water, lukewarm 80° F

· 1 teaspoon table salt

· 4 2/3 cups white bread flour

· 2 2/3 teaspoons bread machine yeast or rapid rise yeast

· 2 baguettes of ¾-pound each

· 1¼ cups water, lukewarm 80° F

· ¾ teaspoon table salt

· 3½ cups white bread flour

· 2 teaspoons bread machine yeast or rapid rise yeast

Other Ingredients:

· Cornmeal

· Olive oil

· 1 egg white

· 1 tablespoon water

Directions:

1.Choose the size of crusty bread you would like to make and measure your ingredients.

2.Add the ingredients for the bread machine to the pan in the order listed above.

3.Put the pan in the bread machine and close the lid. Switch on the bread maker. Select the dough setting.

4.When the dough cycle is completed, remove the pan and lay the dough on a floured working surface.

5.Knead the dough a few times and add flour if needed, so it is not too sticky to handle. Cut the dough in half and form a ball with each half.

6. Grease a baking sheet with olive oil. Dust lightly with cornmeal.

7.Preheat the oven to 375 degrees F and place the oven rack in the middle position.

8.Using a rolling pin dusted with flour, roll one of the dough balls into a 1½ -inch by 9 -inch rectangle for the 2 pounds bread size or a 1¼ -inch by 1 ½ -inch rectangle for the 1½ pound bread size. Starting on the longer side, roll the dough tightly. Pinch the ends and the seam with your fingers to seal. Roll the dough in a back in forth movement to make it into an excellent French baguette shape.

9.Repeat the process with the second dough ball.

10. Place loaves of bread onto the baking sheet with the seams down and brush with some olive oil with enough space in between them to rise. Dust top of both loaves with a little bit of

cornmeal. Cover with a clean towel and place in a warm area with any air draught. Let rise for 5 to 15 minutes, or until loaves doubled in size.

11. Mix the egg white and one tablespoon of water and lightly brush over both loaves of bread.

12. Place in the oven and bake for 1 minute. Remove from oven and brush with remaining egg wash on top of both loaves of bread. Place back into the range, taking care of turning around the baking sheet. Bake for another 5 minutes or until the baguettes are golden brown. Let rest on a wired rack for 5 minutes before serving.

Nutrition:

· Calories: 180

· Fat 0.1½ g

· Carbohydrates: 11 g

· Sodium: 192 mg

· Protein: 3.4 g

Oat Molasses Bread

Preparation Time: 25 minutes

2-Pound Loaf

Ingredients:

· 5 slices bread (2 pounds)

· 1 1/3 cups boiling water

· ¾ cup old-fashioned oats

· 3 tablespoons butter

· 1 large egg, lightly beaten

· 2 teaspoons salt

· ¼ cup honey

· 1½ tablespoons dark molasses

· 4 cups white bread flour

· 2½ teaspoons bread machine yeast

· 1 ½ slice bread (1½ pounds)

· 1 cup boiling water

· ½ cup old-fashioned oats

· 2 tablespoons butter

· 1 large egg, lightly beaten

- 1½ teaspoons table salt

- 3 tablespoons honey

- 1 tablespoon dark molasses

- 3 cups white bread flour

- 2 teaspoons bread machine yeast

Directions:

1.Add the boiling water and oats to a mixing bowl. Allow the oats to soak well and cool down completely. Do not drain the water.

2.Choose the size of bread you would like to make, then measure your ingredients.

3.Add the soaked oats, along with any remaining water, to the bread pan.

4.Put the remaining ingredients in the bread pan in the order listed above.

5.Place the pan in the bread machine, then cover.

6.Press on the machine. Select the Basic setting, then the pound size, and finally, the crust colour. Start the cycle.

7.When the process is finished, then when the bread is baked, remove the pan. Use a potholder as the handle. Rest for a while

8.Take out the bread from the pan and place it in a wire rack. Let it cool for at least 1 minute before slicing.

Nutrition:

· Calories: 187

· Fat: 7.1 g

· Carbohydrates: 11 g

· Sodium: 434 mg

· Protein: 5.1 g

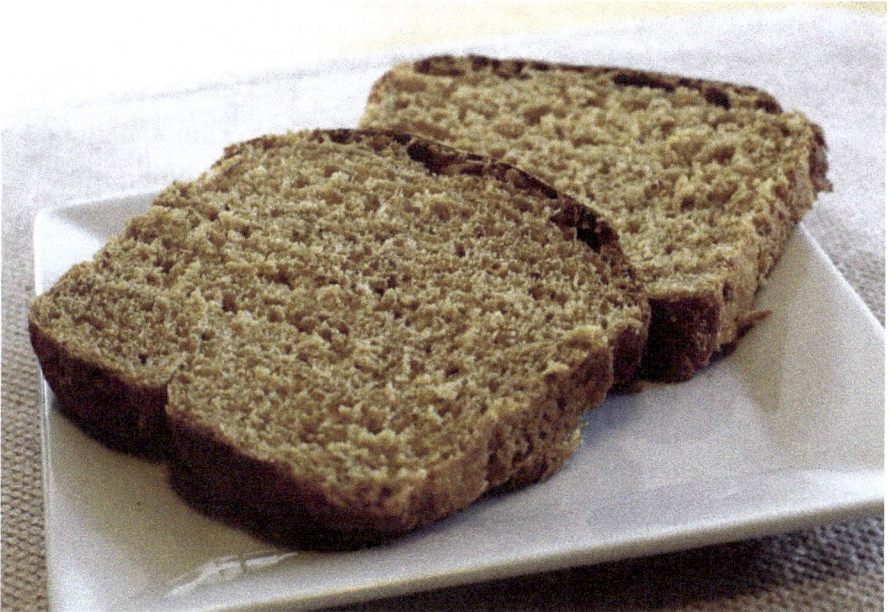

English muffin Bread

Preparation time: 10 minutes

Servings: 14

1- Pound Loaf

Ingredients:

· 1 teaspoon vinegar

· ¼ to 1/3 cup water

· 1 cup lukewarm milk

· 2 tablespoons butter or 2 tablespoons vegetable oil

· 1½ teaspoons salt

· 1½ teaspoons sugar

· ½ teaspoon baking powder

· 3½ cups unbleached all-purpose flour

· 2¼ teaspoons instant yeast

Directions:

1.Add each ingredient to the bread machine in the order and at the temperature recommended by your bread machine manufacturer.

2.Close the lid, select the basic bread, low crust setting on your bread machine, and press start.

3.When the bread machine has finished baking, remove the bread and put it on a cooling rack.

Nutrition:

· Calories: 262

· Carbohydrates: 13 g

· Fat: 1 g

· Protein: 2 g

· Sodium: 360 mg

Whole Wheat Corn Bread

Preparation Time: 2 hours

1 Pound Loaf

Ingredients:

· 5 slices bread (2 pounds)

· 1 1/3 cups lukewarm water

· 2 tablespoons light brown sugar

· 1 large egg, beaten

· 2 tablespoons unsalted butter, melted

· 1½ teaspoons table salt

· ¾ cup whole wheat flour

· ¾ cup cornmeal

· 2¾ cups white bread flour

· 2½ teaspoons bread machine yeast

· 1½ slices bread (1½ pounds)

· 1 cup lukewarm water

· 1½ tablespoons light brown sugar

· 1 medium egg, beaten

· 1½ tablespoons unsalted butter, melted

- 1½ teaspoons table salt

- ½ cup whole wheat flour

- ½ cup cornmeal

- 2 cups of white bread flour

- 1½ teaspoons bread machine yeast

Directions:

1.Choose the size of pound you would like to make and measure your ingredients.

2.Put the ingredients in a pan in the order list above.

3.Put the pan in the bread machine and cover it.

4.Switch on the bread maker. Select the Basic setting, then the pound size, and finally, the crust colour. Start the process.

5.When the process is finished, when the bread is baked, remove the pan from the machine. Use a potholder as the handle. Rest for a while.

6.Take out the bread from the pan and allow to cool on a wire rack for at least 1 minute before slicing.

Nutrition:

- Calories: 194

- Fat: 5.7 g

- Carbohydrates: 19.3 g

Wheat Bran Bread

Preparation Time: 10 minutes

1-Pound Loaf

Ingredients :

· 5 slices bread (2 pounds)

· 1½ cups lukewarm milk

· 3 tablespoons unsalted butter, melted

· ¼ cup of sugar

· 2 teaspoons table salt

· ½ cup wheat bran

· 3½ cups white bread flour

· 2 teaspoons bread machine yeast

· 1½ slices bread (1½ pounds)

· 1½ cups lukewarm milk

· 2¼ tablespoons unsalted butter, melted

· 3 tablespoons sugar

· 1½ teaspoons table salt

· 1/3 cup wheat bran

· 22 /3 cups of white bread flour

· 1½ teaspoons bread machine yeast

Directions:

1.Choose the size of pound you would like to make and measure your ingredients.

2.Put the ingredients into the bread pan in the order listed above.

3.Put the pan in the bread machine and close the lid.

4.Switch on the bread maker. Select the Basic setting, then the pound size, and finally, the crust colour. Start the process.

5.When the process is finished, and the bread is baked, remove the pan from the machine. Use a potholder as the handle. Rest for a few minutes.

6.Take out the bread from the pan and allow to cool on a wire rack for at least 1 minute before slicing.

Nutrition:

· Calories: 184

· Fat: 2.1 g

· Carbohydrates: 24.6 g

· Sodium: 332 mg

Brown & White Sugar Bread

Preparation Time: 10 minutes

1½-Pound Loaf

Ingredients:

· 1 cup milk (room temperature)

· ¼ cup butter, softened

· 1 egg

· ¼ cup light brown sugar

· ¼ cup granulated white sugar

· 2 tablespoons ground cinnamon

· ¼ teaspoon salt

· 3 cups bread flour

· 2 teaspoons bread machine yeast

Directions:

1. Place all ingredients in the baking pan of the bread machine in the order recommended by the manufacturer.

2. Place the baking pan in the bread machine and close the lid.

3. Select Sweet Bread setting and then Medium Crust.

4. Press the start button.

5. Carefully, remove the baking pan from the machine and then invert the bread pound onto a wire rack to cool completely before slicing.

6. With a sharp knife, cut bread pound into desired-sized pounds and serve.

Nutrition:

· Calories: 195

· Total Fat: 5 g

· Saturated Fat: 2.1½ g

· Cholesterol: 25 mg

· Sodium: 94 mg

· Carbohydrates: 33.2 g

· Fiber: 1.6 g

· Sugar: 1½ g

· Protein: 4.7 g

Molasses Bread

Preparation Time: 10 minutes

1½-Pound Loaf

Ingredients:

· 1/3 cup milk

· ¼ cup water

· 3 tablespoons molasses

· 3 tablespoons butter, softened

· 2 cups bread flour

· 1¾ cups whole-wheat flour

· 2 tablespoons white sugar

· 1 teaspoon salt

· 2¼ teaspoons quick-rising yeast

Directions:

1.Place all ingredients in the baking pan of the bread machine in the order recommended by the manufacturer. Place the baking pan in the bread machine and close the lid. Select light browning setting. Press the start button. Carefully, remove the baking pan from the machine and then invert the bread pound onto a wire rack to cool completely before slicing.

2.With a sharp knife, cut bread pound into desired-sized pounds and serve.

Nutrition:

· Calories: 250

· Total Fat: 3.9 g

· Saturated Fat: 1.9 g

· Cholesterol: 1 mg

· Sodium: 240 mg

· Carbohydrates: 37.4 g

· Fiber: 3.1 g

· Sugar: 5.1 g

· Protein: 5.6 g

Honey Bread

Preparation Time: 10 minutes

1-Pound Loaf

Ingredients:

· 1 cup plus 1 tablespoon milk

· 3 tablespoons honey

· 3 tablespoons butter, melted

· 3 cups bread flour

· 1½ teaspoons salt

· 2 teaspoons active dry yeast

Directions:

1.Place all ingredients in the baking pan of the bread machine in the order recommended by the manufacturer.

2.Place the baking pan in the bread machine and close the lid.

3.Select White Bread setting and then Medium Crust.

4.Press the start button.

5.Carefully, remove the baking pan from the machine and then invert the bread pound onto a wire rack to cool completely before slicing.

6. With a sharp knife, cut bread pound into desired-sized pounds and serve.

Nutrition:

· Calories: 176

· Total Fat: 2.7 g

· Saturated Fat: 1.6 g

· Cholesterol: 70 mg

· Sodium: 441 mg

· Carbohydrates: 22.1 g

· Fiber: 0.1½ g

· Sugar: 4 g

· Protein: 3.2 g

Maple Syrup Bread

Preparation Time: 10 minutes

1½-Pound Loaf

Ingredients:

· 1 cup buttermilk

· 2 tablespoons maple syrup

· 2 tablespoons vegetable oil

· 2 tablespoons non-fat dry milk powder

· 1 cup whole-wheat flour

· 2 cups bread flour

· 1 teaspoon salt

· 1½ teaspoons bread machine yeast

Directions:

1.Place all ingredients in the baking pan of the bread machine in the order recommended by the manufacturer.

2.Place the baking pan in the bread machine and close the lid.

3.Select Basic setting.

4.Press the start button.

5.Carefully, remove the baking pan from the machine and then invert the bread pound onto a wire rack to cool completely before slicing.

6. With a sharp knife, cut bread pound into desired-sized pounds and serve.

Nutrition:

· Calories: 171

· Total Fat: 2.6 g

· Saturated Fat: 0.6 g

· Cholesterol: 1 mg

· Sodium: 240 mg

· Total Carbohydrates: 26.1 g

· Fiber: 0.4 g

· Sugar: 3.1½ g

· Protein: 4.7 g

Peanut Butter & Jelly Bread

Preparation Time: 10 minutes

1½-Pound Loaf

Ingredients:

· 1 cup water

· 1½ tablespoons vegetable oil

· ½ cup peanut butter

· ½ cup blackberry jelly

· 1 tablespoon white sugar

· 1 teaspoon salt

· 1 cup whole-wheat flour

· 2 cups bread flour

· 1½ teaspoons active dry yeast

Directions:

1.Place all ingredients in the baking pan of the bread machine in the order recommended by the manufacturer.

2.Place the baking pan in the bread machine and close the lid.

3.Select Sweet Bread setting.

4.Press the start button.

5.Carefully, remove the baking pan from the machine and then invert the bread pound onto a wire rack to cool completely before slicing.

6.With a sharp knife, cut bread pound into desired-sized pounds and serve.

Nutrition:

· Calories: 211

· Total Fat: 7.2 g

· Saturated Fat: 1.5 g

· Cholesterol: 0 mg

· Sodium: 240 mg

· Carbohydrates: 31.6 g

· Fiber: 1.1 g

· Sugar: 2.7 g

· Protein: 6.7 g

Raisin Bread

Preparation Time: 10 minutes

1½-Pound Loaf

Ingredients:

· 1 cup water

· 2 tablespoons margarine

· 3 cups bread flour

· 3 tablespoons white sugar

· 1 teaspoon salt

· 1 teaspoon ground cinnamon

· 2½ teaspoons active dry yeast

· ¾ cup golden raisins

Directions:

1.Place all ingredients (except for raisins) in the baking pan of the bread machine in the order recommended by the manufacturer.

2.Place the baking pan in the bread machine and close the lid.

3.Select Sweet Bread setting.

4.Press the start button.

5.Wait for the bread machine to beep before adding the raisins.

6.Carefully, remove the baking pan from the machine and then invert the bread pound onto a wire rack to cool completely before slicing.

7.With a sharp knife, cut bread pound into desired-sized pounds and serve.

Nutrition:

· Calories: 182

· Total Fat: 2.3 g

· Saturated Fat: 0.4 g

· Cholesterol: 0 mg

· Sodium: 240 mg

· Carbohydrates: 34.5 g

· Fiber: 1.5 g Sugar:11 g

· Protein: 3.9 g

Currant Bread

Preparation Time: 10 minutes

1-Pound Loaf

Ingredients:

· 1¼ cups warm milk

· 2 tablespoons light olive oil

· 2 tablespoons maple syrup

· 3 cups bread flour

· 2 teaspoons ground cardamom

· 1 teaspoon salt

· 2 teaspoons active dry yeast

· ½ cup currants

· ½ cup cashews, chopped finely

Directions:

1.Place all ingredients (except for currants and cashews) in the baking pan of the bread machine in the order recommended by the manufacturer.

2.Place the baking pan in the bread machine and close the lid.

3.Select Basic setting. Press the start button.

4.Wait for the bread machine to beep before adding the currants and cashews.

5.Carefully, remove the baking pan from the machine and then invert the bread pound onto a wire rack to cool completely before slicing.

6. With a sharp knife, cut bread pound into desired-sized pounds and serve.

Nutrition:

· Calories: 232

· Total Fat: 7.1 g

· Saturated Fat: 1.5 g

· Cholesterol: 3 mg

· Sodium: 160 mg

· Carbohydrates: 36.4 g

· Fiber: 1.7 g

· Sugar: 4.6 g

· Protein: 6.4 g

Pineapple Juice Bread

Preparation Time: 10 minutes

1-Pound Loaf

Ingredients:

· ¾ cup fresh pineapple juice

· 1 egg

· 2 tablespoons vegetable oil

· 2½ tablespoons honey

· ¾ teaspoon salt

· 3 cups bread flour

· 2 tablespoons dry milk powder

· 2 teaspoons quick-rising yeast

Directions:

1.Place all ingredients in the baking pan of the bread machine in the order recommended by the manufacturer.

2.Place the baking pan in the bread machine and close the lid.

3.Select Sweet Bread setting and then Light Crust.

4.Press the start button.

5.Carefully, remove the baking pan from the machine and then invert the bread pound onto a wire rack to cool completely before slicing.

6. With a sharp knife, cut bread pound into desired-sized pounds and serve.

Nutrition:

· Calories: 211

· Total Fat: 3 g

· Saturated

· Fat: 0.6 g

· Cholesterol: 1 mg

· Sodium: 180 mg

· Carbohydrates: 30.5

· Fiber: 1 g

· Sugar: 5.9 g

· Protein: 4.5 g

Mocha Bread

Preparation Time: 1 hour

1½-Pound Loaf

Ingredients:

· 1½ cups coffee-flavored liqueur

· ¼ cup water

· 1 (5-ounces) can evaporated milk

· 1 teaspoon salt

· 1½ teaspoons vegetable oil

· 3 cups bread flour

· 2 tablespoons brown sugar

· 1 teaspoon active dry yeast

· ¼ cup semi-sweet mini chocolate chips

Directions:

1.Put ingredients (except the chocolate chips) in the baking pan of the bread machine in the order recommended by the manufacturer.

2.Place the baking pan in the bread machine and close the lid.

3.Select Dough cycle.

4.Press the start button.

5.After the Dough cycle completes, remove the dough from the bread pan and place onto lightly floured surface.

6.With a plastic wrap, cover the dough for about 10 minutes.

7.Uncover the dough and roll it into a rectangle.

8.Sprinkle the dough with chocolate chips and then shape it into a pound.

9.Now, place the dough into a greased pound pan.

10. With a plastic wrap, cover the pound pan and set it in a warm place for 45 minutes or until doubled in size.

11. Preheat your oven to 375°F.

12. Bake for approximately 24–30 minutes or until a wooden skewer inserted in the center comes out clean.

13. Remove the pound pan out of the oven and place onto a wire rack to cool for about 15 minutes.

14. Now, invert bread onto the wire rack to chill completely before slicing.

15. With a sharp knife, cut the bread pound into desired-sized pounds and serve.

Nutrition:

· Calories: 179

· Total Fat: 4.6 g

· Saturated Fat: 1.1 ½ g

· Cholesterol: 3 mg

· Sodium: 240 mg

· Carbohydrates: 29 g

· Fiber: 1.2 g

· Sugars: 5.3 g

· Protein: 4.2 g

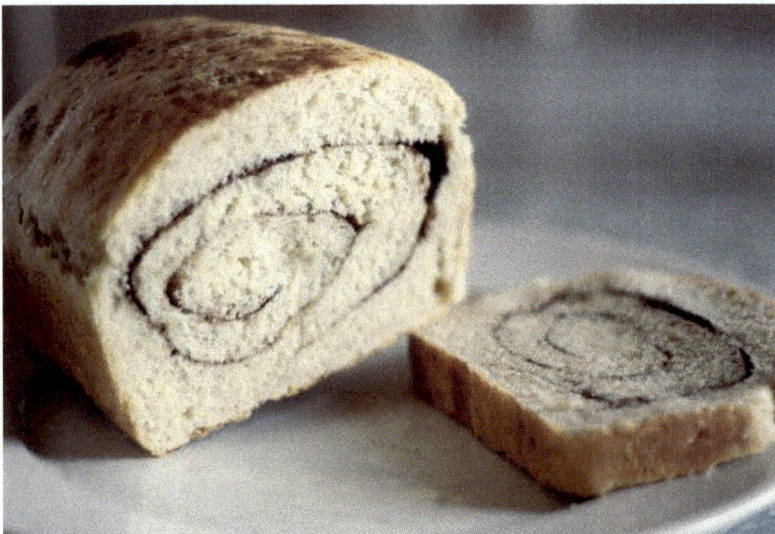

Buttery Sweet Bread

Preparation Time: 10 minutes

1-Pound Loaf

Ingredients:

· 1/3 cup water

· ½ cup milk

· ¼ cup of sugar

· 1 beaten egg

· 1 teaspoon salt

· ¼ cup margarine or ¼ cup butter

· 2 teaspoons bread machine yeast

· 3 1/3 cups bread flour

Directions:

1.Put everything in your bread machine pan.

2.Select the white bread setting.

3.Take out the pan when done and set aside for 11 minutes.

Nutrition:

· Calories: 191

· Carbohydrates: 21½ g

· Total Fat: 5g

· Cholesterol: 0mg

· Protein: 4g

· Fiber: 1g

· Sugars: 3g

· Sodium: 240 mg

· Potassium: 50mg

Cinnamon Sugar Bread

Preparation Time: 10 minutes

1-Pound Loaf

Ingredients:

· ¼ cup margarine or ¼ cup softened butter

· 1 cup milk

· 3 cups of bread flour

· 1 egg

· ½ teaspoon of salt

· ½ cup of sugar

· 2 teaspoons of yeast

· 5 teaspoons of cinnamon

Directions:

1.Put everything in the pan of your bread machine.

2.Select the white bread setting.

3.Take it out when done and set aside for 5 minutes on a rack.

Nutrition:

· Calories: 210

· Carbohydrates: 21 g

· Total Fat: 5g

· Cholesterol: 0 mg

· Protein: 4 g

· Fiber: 1 g

· Sugars 3 g

· Sodium: 122 mg

· Potassium:50 mg

Chocolate Bread

Preparation Time: 10 minutes

1-Pound Loaf

Ingredients:

· 1 pack active dry yeast

· ½ cup of sugar

· 3 cups bread flour

· ¼ cup cocoa powder

· 1 large egg

· ¼ cup butter

· ½ teaspoon vanilla extract

· 1 cup milk

Directions:

1.Put everything in the pan of your bread machine.

2.Select the quick bread or equivalent setting.

3.Take out the pan when done and set aside for 5minutes.

Nutrition:

· Calories: 214

· Carbohydrates: 31 g

· Total Fat: 5 g

· Cholesterol: 13 mg

· Protein: 5 g

· Fiber: 2 g

· Sugars: 1½ g

· Sodium: 21 mg

· Potassium: 92 mg

Cranberry Walnut Bread

Preparation Time: 10 minutes

Ingredients:

· ¼ cup of water

· ¼ cup rolled oats

· 1 egg

· 1 cup buttermilk

· 1½ tablespoons margarine

· 3 tablespoons honey

· 1 teaspoon salt

· 3 cups bread flour

· ½ teaspoon ground cinnamon

· ¼ teaspoon baking soda

· ¾ cup dried cranberries

· 2 teaspoons active dry yeast

· ½ cup chopped walnuts

Directions:

1.Put everything in your bread machine pan, except the walnuts and cranberries.

2.Set the machine to the light crust and the sweet cycle modes.

3. Hit the start button.

4.Add the walnuts and cranberries at the beep signal.

5.Take out the pan when done and set aside for 5minutes.

Nutrition:

· Calories: 210

· Carbohydrates: 31 g

· Total Fat: 5 g

· Cholesterol: 13 mg

· Protein: 5 g

· Fiber: 2 g

· Sugar 1½ g

· Sodium: 240 mg

· Potassium: 92 mg

Coconut Ginger Bread

Preparation Time: 10 minutes

1-Pound Loaf

Ingredients:

· 1 cup + 2 tablespoons Half & Half

· 1¼ cups toasted shredded coconut

· 2 large eggs

· ¼ cup oil

· 1 teaspoon coconut extract

· 1 teaspoon lemon extract

· ¾ cup sugar

· 1 tablespoon grated lemon peel

· 2 cups all-purpose flour

· 2 tablespoons finely chopped candied ginger

· 1 teaspoon baking powder

· ½ teaspoon salt

· 1¼ cups toasted shredded coconut

Directions:

1.Put everything in your bread machine pan.

2.Select the quick bread mode.

3.Press the start button.

4.Allow bread to cool on the wire rack until ready to serve (at least 1 minute).

Nutrition:

· Calories: 210

· Carbohydrates: 45 g

· Total Fat: 3 g

· Cholesterol: 3 mg

· Protein: 5 g

· Fiber: 2 g

· Sugar 15 g

· Sodium: 120 mg

· Potassium: 61 mg

Hawaiian Sweet Bread

Preparation Time: 10 minutes

1-Pound Loaf

Ingredients:

· ¾ cup pineapple juice

· 1 egg

· 2 tablespoons vegetable oil

· 2 ½ tablespoons honey

· ¾ teaspoon salt

· 3 cups bread flour 2

· 2 tablespoons dry milk

· 2 teaspoons fast-rising yeast

Directions:

1.Place ingredients in bread machine container.

2.Select the white bread cycle.

3.Press the start button.

4.Take out the pan when done and set aside for 5minutes.

Nutrition:

· Calories: 249

· Carbohydrates: 25 g

· Total Fat: 5 g

· Cholesterol: 25 mg

· Protein: 4 g

· Fiber: 1 g

· Sugars: 5 g

· Sodium: 180 mg

· Potassium: 76 mg

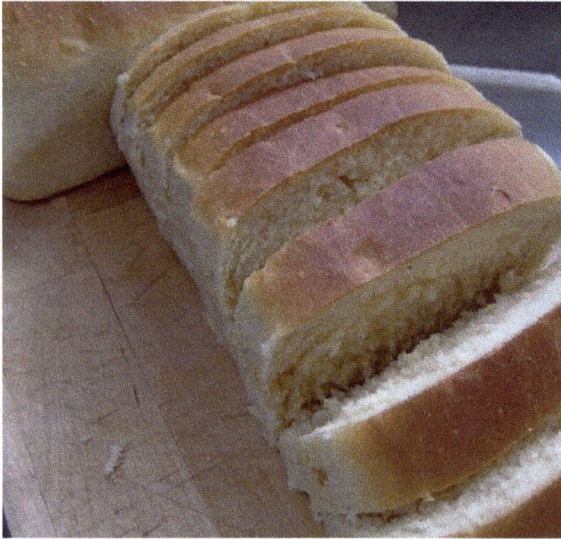

Easy Donuts

Preparation Time: 1 hour

1½-Pound Loaf

Ingredients:

· 2/3 cup milk, room temperature

· ¼ cup water, room temperature

· ½ cup of warm water

· ¼ cup softened butter

· 1 egg slightly has beaten

· ¼ cup granulated sugar

· 1 teaspoon salt

· 3 cups bread machine flour

· 2½ teaspoons bread machine yeast

· oil for deep frying

· ¼ cup confectioners sugar

Directions:

1.Place the milk, water, butter, egg, sugar, salt, flour, and yeast in a pan.

2.Select dough setting and push start. Press the start button.

3.When the process is complete, remove dough from the pan and transfer it to a lightly floured surface.

4. Using a rolling pin lightly dusted with flour, roll dough to ½ inch thickness.

5.Cut with a floured dusted donut cutter or circle cookie cutter.

6.Transfer donuts to a baking sheet that has been covered with wax paper. Place another layer of paper on top, then cover with a clean tea towel. Let rise 30-40 minutes.

7.Heat vegetable oil to 375° F (190° C) in a deep-fryer or large, heavy pot.

8.Fry donuts 2-3 at a time until golden brown on both sides for about 3 minutes.

9.Drain on a paper towel.

10. Sprinkle with confectioners' sugar.

Nutrition:

· Calories: 220

· Carbohydrates: 30 g

· Total Fat: 5 g

· Cholesterol: 25 mg

· Protein: 4 g

· Fiber: 2 g

Date and Nut Bread

Preparation Time: 10 minutes

1-Pound Loaf

Ingredients:

· 1½ tablespoons vegetable oil

· 1 cup of water

· ½ teaspoon salt

· 2 tablespoons honey

· ¾ cup whole-wheat flour

· ¾ cup rolled oats

· 1½ teaspoons active dry yeast

· 1½ cups bread flour

· ½ cup almonds, chopped

· ½ cup dates, chopped and pitted

Directions:

1.Put everything in your bread machine pan.

2.Select the primary cycle. Press the start button.

3.Take out the pan when done and set aside for 5minutes.

Nutrition:

· Calories: 222

· Carbohydrates: 17 g

· Fat: 5g

· Cholesterol: 0 mg

· Protein: 3 g

· Fiber: 3 g

· Sugar: 7 g

· Sodium: 120 mg

· Potassium: 130 mg

Pumpkin Bread

Preparation Time: 10 minutes

1-Pound Loaf

Ingredients:

- ½ cup plus 2 tablespoons warm water
- ½ cup canned pumpkin puree
- ¼ cup butter, softened
- ¼ cup non-fat dry milk powder
- 2 ¾ cups bread flour
- ¼ cup brown sugar
- ¾ teaspoon salt
- 1 teaspoon ground cinnamon
- ½ teaspoon ground ginger
- 1½ teaspoons ground nutmeg
- 2¼ teaspoons active dry yeast

Directions:

1.Place all ingredients in the baking pan of the bread machine in the order recommended by the manufacturer.

2.Place the baking pan in the bread machine and close the lid.

3.Select Basic setting.

4.Press the start button.

5.Carefully, remove the baking pan from the machine and then invert the bread pound onto a wire rack to cool completely before slicing.

6.With a sharp knife, cut bread pound into desired-sized pounds and serve.

Nutrition:

· Calories: 184

· Total Fat 3.6 g

· Saturated Fat: 2.1 g

· Cholesterol: 9 mg

· Sodium: 180 mg

· Carbohydrates: 22.4 g

· Fiber: 1.1 g

· Sugars: 2.9 g

· Protein: 2.9 g

Pumpkin Cranberry Bread

Preparation Time: 15 minutes

1½-Pound Loaf

Ingredients:

· ¾ cup water

· 2/3 cup canned pumpkin

· 3 tablespoons brown sugar

· 2 tablespoons vegetable oil

· 2 cups all-purpose flour

· 1 cup whole-wheat flour

· 1¼ teaspoons salt

· ½ cup sweetened dried cranberries

· ½ cup walnuts, chopped

· 1¾ teaspoons active dry yeast

Directions:

1.Place all ingredients in the baking pan of the bread machine in the order recommended by the manufacturer.

2.Place the baking pan in the bread machine and close the lid.

3.Select Basic setting.

4.Press the start button.

5. Carefully, remove the baking pan from the machine and then invert the bread pound onto a wire rack to cool completely before slicing.

6.With a sharp knife, cut bread pound into desired-sized pounds and serve.

Nutrition:

· Calories: 199

· Total Fat: 6 g

· Saturated Fat: 0.7 g

· Cholesterol: 0 mg

· Sodium: 320 mg

· Carbohydrates: 31.4 g

· Fiber: 3.2 g

· Sugars: 5.1 g

· Protein: 5.6 g

Cranberry Bread

Preparation Time: 15 minutes

1-pound Loaf

Ingredients:

· 1 cup plus 3 tablespoons water

· ¼ cup honey

· 2 tablespoons butter, softened

· 4 cups bread flour

· 1 teaspoon salt

· 2 teaspoons bread machine yeast

· ¾ cup dried cranberries

Directions:

1. Place all ingredients (except the cranberries) in the baking pan of the bread machine in the order recommended by the manufacturer.

2. Place the baking pan in the bread machine and close the lid.

3. Select sweet bread setting.

4. Press the start button.

5.Wait for the bread machine to beep before adding the cranberries.

6.Carefully, remove the baking pan from the machine and then invert the bread pound onto a wire rack to cool completely before slicing.

7.With a sharp knife, cut bread pound into desired-sized pounds and serve.

Nutrition:

· Calories: 233

· Total Fat: 1.1 g

· Saturated Fat: 1 g

· Cholesterol: 4 mg

· Sodium: 240 mg

· Carbohydrates: 21 g

· Fiber: 1.2 g

· Sugars: 4.6 g

· Protein: 3.5 g

Cranberry Orange Bread

Preparation Time: 15 minutes

1½-Pound Loaf

Ingredients:

· 3 cups all-purpose flour

· 1 cup dried cranberries

· ¾ cup plain yogurt

· ½ cup warm water

· 3 tablespoons honey

· 1 tablespoon butter, melted

· 2 teaspoons active dry yeast

· 1½ teaspoons salt

· 1 teaspoon orange oil

Directions:

1.Place all ingredients in the baking pan of the bread machine in the order recommended by the manufacturer.

2.Place the baking pan in the bread machine and close the lid.

3.Select Basic setting and then Light Crust.

4.Press the start button.

5.Carefully, remove the baking pan from the machine and then invert the bread pound onto a wire rack to cool completely before slicing.

6.With a sharp knife, cut bread pound into desired-sized pounds and serve.

Nutrition:

· Calories: 246

· Total Fat: 2.7 g

· Saturated Fat: 1 g

· Cholesterol: 3 mg

· Sodium: 360 mg

· Carbohydrates: 30.4 g

· Fiber: 1.3 g

· Sugars: 5.1 g

· Protein: 4.4 g